The Best Air Fryer Cooking Guide

An Unmissable Recipe Collection for Your
Air Fryer Meals

Eva Sheppard

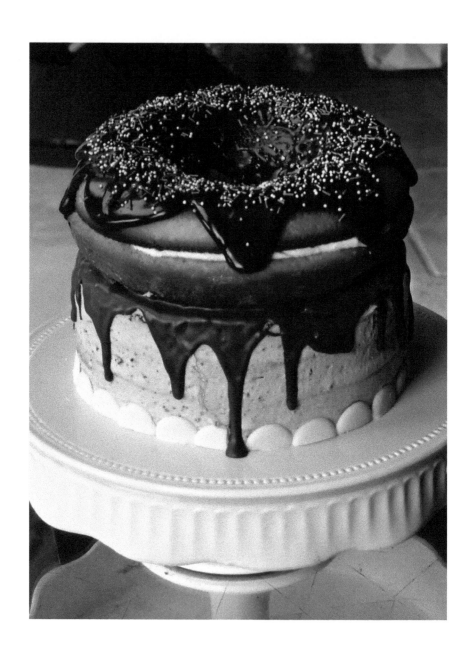

TABLE OF CONTENT

Chili Cheese Balls... 8

Juicy Pickled Chips 10

Coconut Chicken Bites 11

Buffalo Cauliflower Snack.. 13

Banana Snack 16

Potato Spread 18

Mexican Apple Snack 20

Shrimp Muffins.. 22

Zucchini Cakes.. 24

Cauliflower Bars.. 26

Pesto Crackers.. 28

Pumpkin Muffins.. 30

Zucchini Chips... 32

Beef Jerky Snack... 33

Honey Party Wings.. 36

Salmon Party Patties 38

Banana Chips 40

Spring Rolls 42

Easy Cheesecake Recipe 44

Macaroons Recipe... 46

Orange Cake Recipe 47

Bread Dough and Amaretto Dessert Recipe 49

Carrot Cake Recipe *52*

Banana Bread Recipe *54*

Easy Granola Recipe *56*

Pears and Espresso Cream Recipe *58*

Banana Cake Recipe *60*

Fried Bananas Recipe *62*

Coffee Cheesecakes Recipe *64*

Tomato Cake Recipe *66*

Chocolate Cake Recipe *68*

Cinnamon Rolls and Cream Cheese Dip Recipe *70*

Pumpkin Cookies Recipe *72*

Apple Bread Recipe *74*

Strawberry Pie Recipe *76*

Bread Pudding Recipe *78*

Chocolate and Pomegranate Bars Recipe *80*

Lemony Cheesecake *82*

Baked Apples *84*

Dark Chocolate Brownies *85*

Chocolate and Raspberry Cake *87*

Moon Pie *89*

Apple Caramel Relish *91*

Chocolate and Peanut Butter Fondants *93*

White Chocolate Pudding *97*

Lemon Curd *99*

Almond Meringue Cookies *101*

Chocolate Banana Sandwiches *103*

Crème Brulee *105*

The Most Chocolaty Fudge *108*

Chili Cheese Balls

Preparation Time: 50 min

Servings: 6

Nutrition Values: Calories 395; Carbs 45g; Fat 13g; Protein 23g

Ingredients

- 2 cups crumbled Cottage cheese
- 2 cups grated Parmesan cheese
- 2 red potatoes, peeled and chopped
- 1 medium onion, finely chopped
- 1 ½ tsp red chili flakes
- 1 green chili, finely chopped
- Salt to taste
- 4 tbsp chopped coriander leaves
- 1 cup flour
- 1 cup breadcrumbs
- Water

Directions

1. Place the potatoes in a pot, add water and bring them to boil over medium heat for 25 to 30 minutes until soft. Turn off the heat, drain the potatoes through a sieve, and place in a bowl. With a potato masher, mash the potatoes and leave to cool.

2. Add the cottage cheese, Parmesan cheese, onion, red chili flakes, green chili, salt, coriander, and flour to the potato mash. Use a wooden spoon to mix the ingredients well, then, use your hands to mold out bite-size balls. Pour the crumbs in a bowl and roll each cheese ball lightly in it.

3. Place them on a tray. Put 8 to 10 cheese balls in the fryer basket, and cook for 15 minutes at 350 F. Repeat the cooking process for the remaining cheese balls. Serve with tomato-basil dip.

Juicy Pickled Chips

Preparation Time: 20 min

Servings: 3

Nutrition Values: Calories: 140; Carbs: 17g; Fat: 7g; Protein: 2g

Ingredients

- 36 sweet pickle chips
- 1 cup buttermilk
- 3 tbsp smoked paprika
- 2 cups flour
- ¼ cup cornmeal
- Salt and black pepper to taste

Directions

1. Preheat your Air Fryer to 400 F. Using a bowl mix flour, paprika, pepper, salt, cornmeal and powder. Place pickles in buttermilk and set aside for 5 minutes. Dip the pickles in the spice mixture and place them in the air fryer's cooking basket. Cook for 10 minutes.

Coconut Chicken Bites

Preparation time: 10 minutes

Cooking time: 13 minutes

Servings: 4

Ingredients:

- 2 teaspoons garlic powder
- 2 eggs
- Salt and black pepper to the taste
- ¾ cup panko bread crumbs
- ¾ cup coconut, shredded
- Cooking spray
- 8 chicken tenders

Directions:

2. In a bowl, mix eggs with salt, pepper and garlic powder and whisk well.

3. In another bowl, mix coconut with panko and stir well.

4. Dip chicken tenders in eggs mix and then coat in coconut one well.

5. Spray chicken bites with cooking spray, place them in your air fryer's basket and cook them at 350 degrees F for 10 minutes.

6. Arrange them on a platter and serve as an appetizer.

7. Enjoy!

Nutrition Values: calories 252, fat 4, fiber 2, carbs 14, protein 24

Buffalo Cauliflower Snack

Preparation time: 10 minutes

Cooking time: 15 minutes

Servings: 4

Ingredients:

- 4 cups cauliflower florets
- 1 cup panko bread crumbs
- ¼ cup butter, melted
- ¼ cup buffalo sauce
- Mayonnaise for serving

Directions:

1. In a bowl, mix buffalo sauce with butter and whisk well.

2. Dip cauliflower florets in this mix and coat them in panko bread crumbs.

3. Place them in your air fryer's basket and cook at 350 degrees F for 15 minutes.

4. Arrange them on a platter and serve with mayo on the side.

5. Enjoy!

Nutrition Values: calories 241, fat 4, fiber 7, carbs 8, protein 4

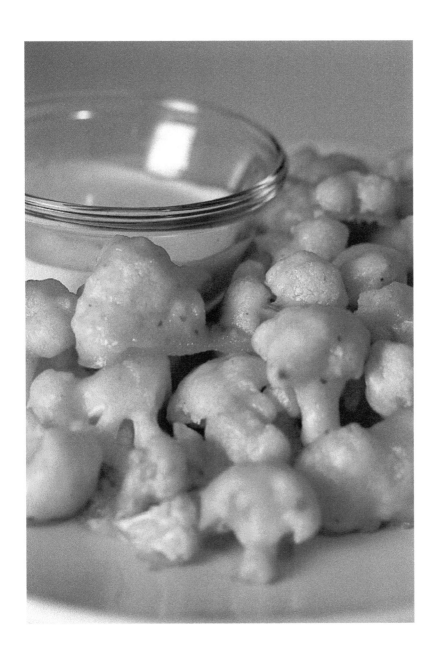

Banana Snack

Preparation time: 10 minutes

Cooking time: 5 minutes

Servings: 8

Ingredients:

- 16 baking cups crust
- ¼ cup peanut butter
- ¾ cup chocolate chips
- 1 banana, peeled and sliced into 16 pieces
- 1 tablespoon vegetable oil

Directions:

1. Put chocolate chips in a small pot, heat up over low heat, stir until it melts and take off heat.

2. In a bowl, mix peanut butter with coconut oil and whisk well.

3. Spoon 1 teaspoon chocolate mix in a cup, add 1 banana slice and top with 1 teaspoon butter mix

4. Repeat with the rest of the cups, place them all into a dish that fits your air fryer, cook at 320 degrees F for 5 minutes, transfer to a freezer and keep there until you serve them as a snack.

5. Enjoy!

Nutrition Values: calories 70, fat 4, fiber 1, carbs 10, protein 1

Potato Spread

Preparation time: 10 minutes

Cooking time: 10 minutes

Servings: 10

Ingredients:

- 19 ounces canned garbanzo beans, drained
- 1 cup sweet potatoes, peeled and chopped
- ¼ cup tahini
- 2 tablespoons lemon juice
- 1 tablespoon olive oil
- 5 garlic cloves, minced
- ½ teaspoon cumin, ground
- 2 tablespoons water
- A pinch of salt and white pepper

Directions:

1. Put potatoes in your air fryer's basket, cook them at 360 degrees F for 15 minutes, cool them down, peel, put them in your food processor and pulse well. basket,

18

2. Add sesame paste, garlic, beans, lemon juice, cumin, water and oil and pulse really well.

3. Add salt and pepper, pulse again, divide into bowls and serve.

4. Enjoy!

Nutrition Values: calories 200, fat 3, fiber 10, carbs 20, protein 11

Mexican Apple Snack

Preparation time: 10 minutes

Cooking time: 5 minutes

Servings: 4

Ingredients:

- 3 big apples, cored, peeled and cubed
- 2 teaspoons lemon juice
- ¼ cup pecans, chopped
- ½ cup dark chocolate chips
- ½ cup clean caramel sauce

Directions:

1. In a bowl, mix apples with lemon juice, stir and transfer to a pan that fits your air fryer.

2. Add chocolate chips, pecans, drizzle the caramel sauce, toss, introduce in your air fryer and cook at 320 degrees F for 5 minutes.

3. Toss gently, divide into small bowls and serve right away as a snack.

4. Enjoy!

Nutrition Values: calories 200, fat 4, fiber 3, carbs 20, protein 3

Shrimp Muffins

Preparation time: 10 minutes

Cooking time: 26 minutes

Servings: 6

Ingredients:

- 1 spaghetti squash, peeled and halved
- 2 tablespoons mayonnaise
- 1 cup mozzarella, shredded
- 8 ounces shrimp, peeled, cooked and chopped
- 1 and ½ cups panko
- 1 teaspoon parsley flakes
- 1 garlic clove, minced
- Salt and black pepper to the taste
- Cooking spray

Directions:

1. Put squash halves in your air fryer, cook at 350 degrees F for 16 minutes, leave aside to cool down and scrape flesh into a bowl.

2. Add salt, pepper, parsley flakes, panko, shrimp, mayo and mozzarella and stir well.

3. Spray a muffin tray that fits your air fryer with cooking spray and divide squash and shrimp mix in each cup.

4. Introduce in the fryer and cook at 360 degrees F for 10 minutes.

5. Arrange muffins on a platter and serve as a snack.

6. Enjoy!

Nutrition Values: calories 60, fat 2, fiber 0.4, carbs 4, protein 4

Zucchini Cakes

Preparation time: 10 minutes

Cooking time: 12 minutes

Servings: 12

Ingredients:

- Cooking spray
- ½ cup dill, chopped
- 1 egg
- ½ cup whole wheat flour
- Salt and black pepper to the taste
- 1 yellow onion, chopped
- 2 garlic cloves, minced
- 3 zucchinis, grated

Directions:

1. In a bowl, mix zucchinis with garlic, onion, flour, salt, pepper, egg and dill, stir well, shape small patties out of this mix, spray them with cooking spray, place them in

your air fryer's basket and cook at 370 degrees F for 6 minutes on each side.

2. Serve them as a snack right away.

3. Enjoy!

Nutrition Values: calories 60, fat 1, fiber 2, carbs 6, protein 2

Cauliflower Bars

Preparation time: 10 minutes

Cooking time: 25 minutes

Servings: 12

Ingredients:

- 1 big cauliflower head, florets separated

- ½ cup mozzarella, shredded

- ¼ cup egg whites

- 1 teaspoon Italian seasoning

- Salt and black pepper to the taste

Directions:

1. Put cauliflower florets in your food processor, pulse well, spread on a lined baking sheet that fits your air fryer, introduce in the fryer and cook at 360 degrees F for 10 minutes.

2. Transfer cauliflower to a bowl, add salt, pepper, cheese, egg whites and Italian seasoning, stir really well, spread this into

a rectangle pan that fits your air fryer, press well, introduce in the fryer and cook at 360 degrees F for 15 minutes more.

3. Cut into 12 bars, arrange them on a platter and serve as a snack

4. Enjoy!

Nutrition Values: calories 50, fat 1, fiber 2, carbs 3, protein 3

Pesto Crackers

Preparation time: 10 minutes

Cooking time: 17 minutes

Servings: 6

Ingredients:

- ½ teaspoon baking powder
- Salt and black pepper to the taste
- 1 and ¼ cups flour
- ¼ teaspoon basil, dried
- 1 garlic clove, minced
- 2 tablespoons basil pesto
- 3 tablespoons butter

Directions:

1. In a bowl, mix salt, pepper, baking powder, flour, garlic, cayenne, basil, pesto and butter and stir until you obtain a dough.

2. Spread this dough on a lined baking sheet that fits your air fryer, introduce in the fryer at 325 degrees F and bake for 17 minutes.

3. Leave aside to cool down, cut crackers and serve them as a snack.

4. Enjoy!

Nutrition Values: calories 200, fat 20, fiber 1, carbs 4, protein 7

Pumpkin Muffins

Preparation time: 10 minutes

Cooking time: 15 minutes

Servings: 18

Ingredients:

- ¼ cup butter
- ¾ cup pumpkin puree
- 2 tablespoons flaxseed meal
- ¼ cup flour
- ½ cup sugar
- ½ teaspoon nutmeg, ground
- 1 teaspoon cinnamon powder
- ½ teaspoon baking soda
- 1 egg
- ½ teaspoon baking powder

Directions:

1. In a bowl, mix butter with pumpkin puree and egg and blend well.

2. Add flaxseed meal, flour, sugar, baking soda, baking powder, nutmeg and cinnamon and stir well.

3. Spoon this into a muffin pan that fits your fryer introduce in the fryer at 350 degrees F and bake for 15 minutes.

4. Serve muffins cold as a snack.

5. Enjoy!

Nutrition Values: calories 50, fat 3, fiber 1, carbs 2, protein 2

Zucchini Chips

Preparation time: 10 minutes

Cooking time: 1 hour

Servings: 6

Ingredients:

- 3 zucchinis, thinly sliced
- Salt and black pepper to the taste
- 2 tablespoons olive oil
- 2 tablespoons balsamic vinegar

Directions:

1. In a bowl, mix oil with vinegar, salt and pepper and whisk well.

2. Add zucchini slices, toss to coat well, introduce in your air fryer and cook at 200 degrees F for 1 hour.

3. Serve zucchini chips cold as a snack.

4. Enjoy!

Nutrition Values: calories 40, fat 3, fiber 7, carbs 3, protein 7

Beef Jerky Snack

Preparation time: 2 hours

Cooking time: 1 hour and 30 minutes

Servings: 6

Ingredients:

- 2 cups soy sauce

- ½ cup Worcestershire sauce

- 2 tablespoons black peppercorns

- 2 tablespoons black pepper

- 2 pounds beef round, sliced

Directions:

1. In a bowl, mix soy sauce with black peppercorns, black pepper and Worcestershire sauce and whisk well.

2. Add beef slices, toss to coat and leave aside in the fridge for 6 hours.

3. Introduce beef rounds in your air fryer and cook them at 370 degrees F for 1 hour and 30 minutes.

4. Transfer to a bowl and serve cold.

5. Enjoy!

Nutrition Values: calories 300, fat 12, fiber 4, carbs 3, protein 8

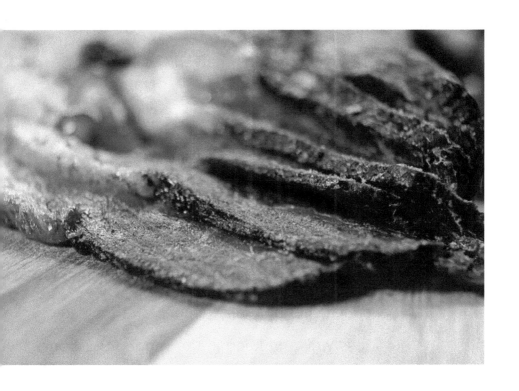

Honey Party Wings

Preparation time: 1 hour and 10 minutes

Cooking time: 12 minutes

Servings: 8

Ingredients:

- 16 chicken wings, halved
- 2 tablespoons soy sauce
- 2 tablespoons honey
- Salt and black pepper to the taste
- 2 tablespoons lime juice

Directions:

1. In a bowl, mix chicken wings with soy sauce, honey, salt, pepper and lime juice, toss well and keep in the fridge for 1 hour.

2. Transfer chicken wings to your air fryer and cook them at 360 degrees F for 12 minutes, flipping them halfway.

3. Arrange them on a platter and serve as an appetizer.

4. Enjoy!

Nutrition Values: calories 211, fat 4, fiber 7, carbs 14, protein 3

Salmon Party Patties

Preparation time: 10 minutes

Cooking time: 22 minutes

Servings: 4

Ingredients:

- 3 big potatoes, boiled, drained and mashed
- 1 big salmon fillet, skinless, boneless
- 2 tablespoons parsley, chopped
- 2 tablespoon dill, chopped
- Salt and black pepper to the taste
- 1 egg
- 2 tablespoons bread crumbs
- Cooking spray

Directions:

1. Place salmon in your air fryer's basket and cook for 10 minutes at 360 degrees F.

2. Transfer salmon to a cutting board, cool it down, flake it and put it in a bowl.

3. Add mashed potatoes, salt, pepper, dill, parsley, egg and bread crumbs, stir well and shape 8 patties out of this mix.

4. Place salmon patties in your air fryer's basket, spry them with cooking oil, cook at 360 degrees F for 12 minutes, flipping them halfway, transfer them to a platter and serve as an appetizer.

5. Enjoy!

Nutrition Values: calories 231, fat 3, fiber 7, carbs 14, protein 4

Banana Chips

Preparation time: 10 minutes

Cooking time: 15 minutes

Servings: 4

Ingredients:

- 4 bananas, peeled and sliced
- A pinch of salt
- ½ teaspoon turmeric powder
- ½ teaspoon chaat masala
- 1 teaspoon olive oil

Directions:

1. In a bowl, mix banana slices with salt, turmeric, chaat masala and oil, toss and leave aside for 10 minutes.

2. Transfer banana slices to your preheated air fryer at 360 degrees F and cook them for 15 minutes flipping them once.

3. Serve as a snack.

4. Enjoy!

Nutrition Values: calories 121, fat 1, fiber 2, carbs 3, protein 3

Spring Rolls

Preparation time: 10 minutes

Cooking time: 25 minutes

Servings: 8

Ingredients:

- 2 cups green cabbage, shredded
- 2 yellow onions, chopped
- 1 carrot, grated
- ½ chili pepper, minced
- 1 tablespoon ginger, grated
- 3 garlic cloves, minced
- 1 teaspoon sugar
- Salt and black pepper to the taste
- 1 teaspoon soy sauce
- 2 tablespoons olive oil
- 10 spring roll sheets
- 2 tablespoons corn flour
- 2 tablespoons water

Directions:

1. Heat up a pan with the oil over medium heat, add cabbage, onions, carrots, chili pepper, ginger, garlic, sugar, salt, pepper and soy sauce, stir well, cook for 2-3 minutes, take off heat and cool down.

2. Cut spring roll sheets in squares, divide cabbage mix on each and roll them.

3. In a bowl, mix corn flour with water, stir well and seal spring rolls with this mix.

4. Place spring rolls in your air fryer's basket and cook them at 360 degrees F for 10 minutes.

5. Flip roll and cook them for 10 minutes more.

6. Arrange on a platter and serve them as an appetizer.

7. Enjoy!

Nutrition Values: calories 214, fat 4, fiber 4, carbs 12, protein 4

Easy Cheesecake Recipe

Preparation Time: 25 Minutes

Servings: 15

Ingredients:

- 1 lb. cream cheese

- 1/2 tsp. vanilla extract

- 1 cup graham crackers; crumbled

- 2 tbsp. butter

- 2 eggs

- 4 tbsp. sugar

Directions:

1. In a bowl; mix crackers with butter.

2. Press crackers mix on the bottom of a lined cake pan, introduce in your air fryer and cook at 350 °F, for 4 minutes

3. Meanwhile; in a bowl, mix sugar with cream cheese, eggs and vanilla and whisk well.

4. Spread filling over crackers crust and cook your cheesecake in your air fryer at 310 °F,

for 15 minutes. Leave cake in the fridge for
3 hours, slice and serve

Nutrition Values: Calories: 245; Fat: 12; Fiber:
1; Carbs: 20; Protein: 3

Macaroons Recipe

Preparation Time: 18 Minutes

Servings: 20

Ingredients:

- 2 tbsp. sugar

- 2 cup coconut; shredded

- 4 egg whites

- 1 tsp. vanilla extract

Directions:

1. In a bowl; mix egg whites with stevia and beat using your mixer

2. Add coconut and vanilla extract, whisk again, shape small balls out of this mix, introduce them in your air fryer and cook at 340 °F, for 8 minutes. Serve macaroons cold

Nutrition Values: Calories: 55; Fat: 6; Fiber: 1; Carbs: 2; Protein: 1

Orange Cake Recipe

Preparation Time: 42 Minutes

Servings: 12

Ingredients:

- 1 orange, peeled and cut into quarters
- 1 tsp. vanilla extract
- 6 eggs
- 2 tbsp. orange zest
- 4 oz. cream cheese
- 1 tsp. baking powder
- 9 oz. flour
- 2 oz. sugar+ 2 tbsp.
- 4 oz. yogurt

Directions:

1. In your food processor, pulse orange very well

2. Add flour, 2 tbsp. sugar, eggs, baking powder, vanilla extract and pulse well again.

3. Transfer this into 2 spring form pans, introduce each in your fryer and cook at 330 °F, for 16 minutes

4. Meanwhile; in a bowl, mix cream cheese with orange zest, yogurt and the rest of the sugar and stir well.

5. Place one cake layer on a plate, add half of the cream cheese mix, add the other cake layer and top with the rest of the cream cheese mix. Spread it well, slice and serve.

Nutrition Values: Calories: 200; Fat: 13; Fiber: 2; Carbs: 9; Protein: 8

Bread Dough and Amaretto Dessert Recipe

Preparation Time: 22 Minutes

Servings: 12

Ingredients:

- 1 lb. bread dough
- 1 cup heavy cream
- 12 oz. chocolate chips
- 1 cup sugar
- 1/2 cup butter; melted
- 2 tbsp. amaretto liqueur

Directions:

1. Roll dough, cut into 20 slices and then cut each slice in halves.

2. Brush dough pieces with butter, sprinkle sugar, place them in your air fryer's basket after you've brushed it some butter, cook them at 350 °F, for 5 minutes; flip them,

cook for 3 minutes more and transfer to a platter

3. Heat up a pan with the heavy cream over medium heat, add chocolate chips and stir until they melt. Add liqueur; stir again, transfer to a bowl and serve bread dippers with this sauce

Nutrition Values: Calories: 200; Fat: 1; Fiber: 0; Carbs: 6; Protein: 6

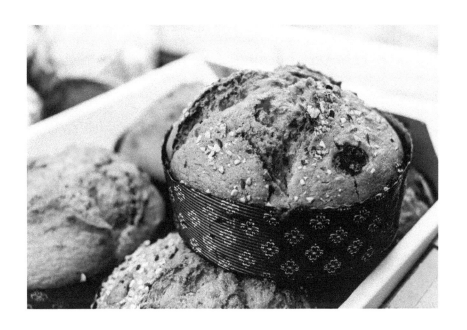

Carrot Cake Recipe

Preparation Time: 55 Minutes

Servings: 6

Ingredients:

- 5 oz. flour

- 3/4 tsp. baking powder

- 1/4 tsp. nutmeg; ground

- 1/2 tsp. baking soda

- 1/2 tsp. cinnamon powder

- 1/2 cup sugar

- 1/3 cup carrots; grated

- 1/3 cup pecans; toasted and chopped.

- 1/4 cup pineapple juice

- 1/2 tsp. allspice

- 1 egg

- 3 tbsp. yogurt

- 4 tbsp. sunflower oil

- 1/3 cup coconut flakes; shredded

- Cooking spray

Directions:

1. In a bowl; mix flour with baking soda and powder, salt, allspice, cinnamon and nutmeg and stir.

2. In another bowl, mix egg with yogurt, sugar, pineapple juice, oil, carrots, pecans and coconut flakes and stir well

3. Combine the two mixtures and stir well, pour this into a spring form pan that fits your air fryer which you've greased with some cooking spray, transfer to your air fryer and cook on 320 °F, for 45 minutes.

4. Leave cake to cool down, then cut and serve it.

Nutrition Values: Calories: 200; Fat: 6; Fiber: 20; Carbs: 22; Protein: 4

Banana Bread Recipe

Preparation Time: 50 Minutes

Servings: 6

Ingredients:

- 3/4 cup sugar

- 1/3 cup butter

- 1/3 cup milk

- 1 tsp. vanilla extract

- 1 egg

- 2 bananas; mashed

- 1 tsp. baking powder

- 1 ½ cups flour

- 1/2 tsp. baking soda

- 1 ½ tsp. cream of tartar

- Cooking spray

Directions:

1. In a bowl; mix milk with cream of tartar, sugar, butter, egg, vanilla and bananas and stir everything.

2. In another bowl, mix flour with baking powder and baking soda

3. Combine the 2 mixtures; stir well, pour this into a cake pan greased with some cooking spray, introduce in your air fryer and cook at 320 °F, for 40 minutes. Take bread out, leave aside to cool down, slice and serve it.

Nutrition Values: Calories: 292; Fat: 7; Fiber: 8; Carbs: 28; Protein: 4

Easy Granola Recipe

Preparation Time: 45 Minutes

Servings: 4

Ingredients:

- 1 cup coconut; shredded

- 1/2 cup almonds

- 1/2 cup pecans; chopped.

- 2 tbsp. sugar

- 1/2 cup pumpkin seeds

- 1/2 cup sunflower seeds

- 2 tbsp. sunflower oil

- 1 tsp. nutmeg; ground

- 1 tsp. apple pie spice mix

Directions:

1. In a bowl; mix almonds and pecans with pumpkin seeds, sunflower seeds, coconut, nutmeg and apple pie spice mix and stir well

2. Heat up a pan with the oil over medium heat, add sugar and stir well.

3. Pour this over nuts and coconut mix and stir well

4. Spread this on a lined baking sheet that fits your air fryer, introduce in your air fryer and cook at 300 °F and bake for 25 minutes. Leave your granola to cool down, cut and serve.

Nutrition Values: Calories: 322; Fat: 7; Fiber: 8; Carbs: 12; Protein: 7

Pears and Espresso Cream Recipe

Preparation Time: 40 Minutes

Servings: 4

Ingredients:

- 4 pears; halved and cored

- 2 tbsp. water

- 2 tbsp. lemon juice

- 1 tbsp. sugar

- 2 tbsp. butter

For the cream:

- 1 cup whipping cream

- 2 tbsp. espresso; cold

- 1 cup mascarpone

- 1/3 cup sugar

Directions:

1. In a bowl; mix pears halves with lemon juice, 1 tbsp. sugar, butter and water, toss

well, transfer them to your air fryer and cook at 360 °F, for 30 minutes

2. Meanwhile; in a bowl, mix whipping cream with mascarpone, ⅓ cup sugar and espresso, whisk really well and keep in the fridge until pears are done.

3. Divide pears on plates, top with espresso cream and serve them

Nutrition Values: Calories: 211; Fat: 5; Fiber: 7; Carbs: 8; Protein: 7

Banana Cake Recipe

Preparation Time: 40 Minutes

Servings: 4

Ingredients:

- 1 tbsp. butter; soft
- 1 egg
- 1/3 cup brown sugar
- 1 tsp. baking powder
- 1/2 tsp. cinnamon powder
- 2 tbsp. honey
- 1 banana; peeled and mashed
- 1 cup white flour
- Cooking spray

Directions:

1. Spray a cake pan with some cooking spray and leave aside.

2. In a bowl; mix butter with sugar, banana, honey, egg, cinnamon, baking powder and flour and whisk

3. Pour this into a cake pan greased with cooking spray, introduce in your air fryer and cook at 350 °F, for 30 minutes. Leave cake to cool down, slice and serve

Nutrition Values: Calories: 232; Fat: 4; Fiber: 1; Carbs: 34; Protein: 4

Fried Bananas Recipe

Preparation Time: 25 Minutes

Servings: 4

Ingredients:

- 3 tbsp. butter

- 3 tbsp. cinnamon sugar

- 1 cup panko

- 2 eggs

- 8 bananas; peeled and halved

- 1/2 cup corn flour

Directions:

1. Heat up a pan with the butter over medium high heat, add panko; stir and cook for 4 minutes and then transfer to a bowl

2. Roll each in flour, eggs and panko mix, arrange them in your air fryer's basket, dust with cinnamon sugar and cook at 280 °F, for 10 minutes. Serve right away.

Nutrition Values: Calories: 164; Fat: 1; Fiber: 4; Carbs: 32; Protein: 4

Coffee Cheesecakes Recipe

Preparation Time: 30 Minutes

Servings: 6

Ingredients:

For the cheesecakes:

- 2 tbsp. butter
- 3 eggs
- 1/3 cup sugar
- 8 oz. cream cheese
- 3 tbsp. coffee
- 1 tbsp. caramel syrup
- For the frosting:
- 3 tbsp. caramel syrup
- 8 oz. mascarpone cheese; soft
- 3 tbsp. butter
- 2 tbsp. sugar

Directions:

1. In your blender, mix cream cheese with eggs, 2 tbsp. butter, coffee, 1 tbsp. caramel syrup and ⅓ cup sugar and pulse very well, spoon into a cupcakes pan that fits your air fryer, introduce in the fryer and cook at 320 °F and bake for 20 minutes

2. Leave aside to cool down and then keep in the freezer for 3 hours. Meanwhile; in a bowl, mix 3 tbsp. butter with 3 tbsp. caramel syrup, 2 tbsp. sugar and mascarpone, blend well, spoon this over cheesecakes and serve them.

Nutrition Values: Calories: 254; Fat: 23; Fiber: 0; Carbs: 21; Protein: 5

Tomato Cake Recipe

Preparation Time: 40 Minutes

Servings: 4

Ingredients:

- 1 ½ cups flour
- 1 tsp. cinnamon powder
- 1 cup tomatoes chopped
- 1/2 cup olive oil
- 1 tsp. baking powder
- 1 tsp. baking soda
- 3/4 cup maple syrup
- 2 tbsp. apple cider vinegar

Directions:

1. In a bowl; mix flour with baking powder, baking soda, cinnamon and maple syrup and stir well.

2. In another bowl, mix tomatoes with olive oil and vinegar and stir well

3. Combine the 2 mixtures; stir well, pour into a greased round pan that fits your air fryer, introduce in the fryer and cook at 360 °F, for 30 minutes. Leave cake to cool down, slice and serve.

Nutrition Values: Calories: 153; Fat: 2; Fiber: 1; Carbs: 25; Protein: 4

Chocolate Cake Recipe

Preparation Time: 40 Minutes

Servings: 12

Ingredients:

- 3/4 cup white flour

- 3/4 cup whole wheat flour

- 1 tsp. baking soda

- 3/4 tsp. pumpkin pie spice

- 3/4 cup sugar

- 1/2 tsp. vanilla extract

- 2/3 cup chocolate chips

- 1 banana; mashed

- 1/2 tsp. baking powder

- 2 tbsp. canola oil

- 1/2 cup Greek yogurt

- 8 oz. canned pumpkin puree

- 1 egg

- Cooking spray

Directions:

1. In a bowl; mix white flour with whole wheat flour, salt, baking soda and powder and pumpkin spice and stir

2. In another bowl, mix sugar with oil, banana, yogurt, pumpkin puree, vanilla and egg and stir using a mixer

3. Combine the 2 mixtures, add chocolate chips; stir, pour this into a greased Bundt pan that fits your air fryer.

4. Introduce in your air fryer and cook at 330 °F, for 30 minutes

5. Leave the cake to cool down, before cutting and serving it.

Nutrition Values: Calories: 232; Fat: 7; Fiber: 7; Carbs: 29; Protein: 4

Cinnamon Rolls and Cream Cheese Dip Recipe

Preparation Time: 2 hours 15 Minutes

Servings: 8

Ingredients:

- 1 lb. bread dough

- 3/4 cup brown sugar

- 1/4 cup butter; melted

- 1 ½ tbsp. cinnamon; ground

- For the cream cheese dip:

- 2 tbsp. butter

- 1 ¼ cups sugar

- 1/2 tsp. vanilla

- 4 oz. cream cheese

Directions:

1. Roll dough on a floured working surface; shape a rectangle and brush with 1/4 cup butter.

2. In a bowl; mix cinnamon with sugar; stir, sprinkle this over dough, roll dough into a log, seal well and cut into 8 pieces

3. Leave rolls to rise for 2 hours, place them in your air fryer's basket, cook at 350 °F, for 5 minutes; flip them, cook for 4 minutes more and transfer to a platter

4. In a bowl; mix cream cheese with butter, sugar and vanilla and whisk really well. Serve your cinnamon rolls with this cream cheese dip.

Nutrition Values: Calories: 200; Fat: 1; Fiber: 0; Carbs: 5; Protein: 6

Pumpkin Cookies Recipe

Preparation Time: 25 Minutes

Servings: 24

Ingredients:

- 2 ½ cups flour
- 1/2 tsp. baking soda
- 2 tbsp. butter
- 1 tsp. vanilla extract
- 1 tbsp. flax seed; ground
- 3 tbsp. water
- 1/2 cup pumpkin flesh; mashed
- 1/4 cup honey
- 1/2 cup dark chocolate chips

Directions:

1. In a bowl; mix flax seed with water; stir and leave aside for a few minutes.

2. In another bowl, mix flour with salt and baking soda

3. In a third bowl, mix honey with pumpkin puree, butter, vanilla extract and flaxseed.

4. Combine flour with honey mix and chocolate chips and stir

5. Scoop 1 tbsp. of cookie dough on a lined baking sheet that fits your air fryer, repeat with the rest of the dough, introduce them in your air fryer and cook at 350 °F, for 15 minutes.

6. Leave cookies to cool down and serve.

Nutrition Values: Calories: 140; Fat: 2; Fiber: 2; Carbs: 7; Protein: 10

Apple Bread Recipe

Preparation Time: 50 Minutes

Servings: 6

Ingredients:

- 3 cups apples; cored and cubed

- 1 cup sugar

- 1 tbsp. baking powder

- 1 stick butter

- 1 tbsp. vanilla

- 2 eggs

- 1 tbsp. apple pie spice

- 2 cups white flour

- 1 cup water

Directions:

1. In a bowl mix egg with 1 butter stick, apple pie spice and sugar and stir using your mixer.

2. Add apples and stir again well

3. In another bowl, mix baking powder with flour and stir.

4. Combine the 2 mixtures; stir and pour into a spring form pan

5. Put spring form pan in your air fryer and cook at 320 °F, for 40 minutes Slice and serve.

Nutrition Values: Calories: 192; Fat: 6; Fiber: 7; Carbs: 14; Protein: 7

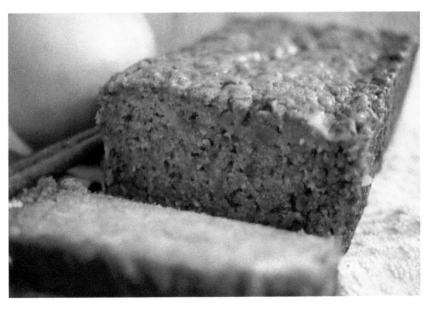

Strawberry Pie Recipe

Preparation Time: 30 Minutes

Servings: 12

Ingredients:

For the crust: y

- 1 cup coconut; shredded
- 1/4 cup butter
- 1 cup sunflower seeds

For the filling:

- 1 tsp. gelatin
- 8 oz. cream cheese
- 1/2 tbsp. lemon juice
- 1/4 tsp. stevia
- 4 oz. strawberries
- 2 tbsp. water
- 1/2 cup heavy cream
- 8 oz. strawberries; chopped for serving

Directions:

1. In your food processor, mix sunflower seeds with coconut, a pinch of salt and butter, pulse and press this on the bottom of a cake pan that fits your air fryer

2. Heat up a pan with the water over medium heat, add gelatin; stir until it dissolves, leave aside to cool down, add this to your food processor, mix with 4 oz. strawberries, cream cheese, lemon juice and stevia and blend well

3. Add heavy cream; stir well and spread this over crust.

4. Top with 8 oz. strawberries, introduce in your air fryer and cook at 330 °F, for 15 minutes. Keep in the fridge until you serve it.

Nutrition Values: Calories: 234; Fat: 23; Fiber: 2; Carbs: 6; Protein: 7

Bread Pudding Recipe

Preparation Time: 1 hour 10 Minutes

Servings: 4

Ingredients:

- 6 glazed doughnuts; crumbled

- 1 cup cherries

- 4 egg yolks

- 1/4 cup sugar

- 1/2 cup chocolate chips.

- 1 ½ cups whipping cream

- 1/2 cup raisins

Directions:

1. In a bowl; mix cherries with egg yolks and whipping cream and stir well.

2. In another bowl, mix raisins with sugar, chocolate chips and doughnuts and stir

3. Combine the 2 mixtures, transfer everything to a greased pan that fits your

air fryer and cook at 310 °F, for 1 hour. Chill
pudding before cutting and serving it

Nutrition Values: Calories: 302; Fat: 8; Fiber:
2; Carbs: 23; Protein: 10

Chocolate and Pomegranate Bars Recipe

Preparation Time: 2 hours 10 Minutes

Servings: 6

Ingredients:

- 1/2 cup milk

- 1/2 cup almonds; chopped

- 1 tsp. vanilla extract

- 1 ½ cups dark chocolate; chopped

- 1/2 cup pomegranate seeds

Directions:

1. Heat up a pan with the milk over medium low heat, add chocolate; stir for 5 minutes; take off heat add vanilla extract, half of the pomegranate seeds and half of the nuts and stir

2. Pour this into a lined baking pan, spread, sprinkle a pinch of salt, the rest of the pomegranate arils and nuts, introduce in

your air fryer and cook at 300 °F, for 4 minutes. Keep in the fridge for 2 hours before serving.

Nutrition Values: Calories: 68; Fat: 1; Fiber: 4; Carbs: 6; Protein: 1

Lemony Cheesecake

Preparation Time: 80 min + chilling time

Servings: 8

Nutrition Values: Calories: 487; Carbs: 23g; Fat: 38g; Protein: 9.3g

Ingredients

- 8 oz graham crackers, crushed
- 4 oz butter, melted
- 16 oz plain cream cheese
- 3 eggs
- 3 tbsp sugar
- 1 tbsp vanilla extract
- Zest of 2 lemons

Directions

1. Line a cake tin, that fits in your Air fryer, with baking paper. Mix together the crackers and butter, and press at the bottom of the tin. In a bowl, add cream cheese, eggs, sugar, vanilla and lemon zest

and beat with a hand mixer until well combined and smooth. Pour the mixture into the tin, on top of the cracker's base. Cook for 40-45 minutes at 350 F, checking it to ensure it's set but still a bit wobbly. Let cool, then refrigerate overnight.

Baked Apples

Preparation Time: 35 min

Servings: 2

Nutrition Values: Calories: 322; Carbs: 37g; Fat: 19g; Protein: 3.8g

Ingredients

- 2 granny smith apples, cored, bottom intact
- 2 tbsp butter, cold
- 3 tbsp sugar
- 3 tbsp crushed walnuts
- 2 tbsp raisins
- 1 tsp cinnamon

Directions

1. In a bowl, add butter, sugar, walnuts, raisins and cinnamon; mix with fingers until you obtain a crumble. Arrange the apples in the Air fryer. Stuff the apples with the filling mixture. Cook for 30 minutes at 400 F.

Dark Chocolate Brownies

Preparation Time: 35 min

Servings: 10

Nutrition Values: Calories: 513; Carbs: 32g; Fat: 55g; Protein: 7g

Ingredients

- 6 oz dark chocolate
- 6 oz butter
- ¾ cup white sugar
- 3 eggs
- 2 tsp vanilla extract
- ¾ cup flour
- ¼ cup cocoa powder
- 1 cup chopped walnuts
- 1 cup white chocolate chips

Directions

1. Line a pan inside your Air fryer with baking paper. In a saucepan, melt chocolate and butter over low heat. Do not stop stirring

until you obtain a smooth mixture. Let cool slightly, whisk in eggs and vanilla. Sift flour and cocoa and stir to mix well. Sprinkle the walnuts over and add the white chocolate into the batter. Pour the batter into the pan and cook for 20 minutes at 340 F. Serve with raspberry syrup and ice cream.

Chocolate and Raspberry Cake

Preparation Time: 40 min

Servings: 8

Nutrition Values: Calories: 486; Carbs: 63g; Fat: 23.6g; Protein: 8.1g

Ingredients

- 1 ½ cups flour
- ⅓ cup cocoa powder
- 2 tsp baking powder
- ¾ cup white sugar
- ¼ cup brown sugar
- ⅔ cup butter
- 2 tsp vanilla extract
- 1 cup milk
- 1 tsp baking soda
- 2 eggs
- 1 cup freeze-dried raspberries
- 1 cup chocolate chips

Directions

1. Line a cake tin with baking powder. In a bowl, sift flour, cocoa and baking powder. Place the sugars, butter, vanilla, milk and baking soda into a microwave-safe bowl and heat for 60 seconds until the butter melts and the ingredients incorporate; let cool slightly. Whisk the eggs into the mixture.

2. Pour the wet ingredients into the dry ones, and fold to combine. Add in the raspberries and chocolate chips into the batter. Pour the batter into the tin and cook for 30 minutes at 350 F.

Moon Pie

Preparation Time: 10 min

Servings: 4

Nutrition Values: Calories: 305; Carbs: 44g; Fat: 13.4g; Protein: 4g

Ingredients

- 4 graham cracker sheets, snapped in half
- 8 large marshmallows
- 8 squares each of dark, milk and white chocolate

Directions

1. Arrange the cracker halves on a board. Put 2 marshmallows onto half of the graham cracker halves. Place 2 squares of chocolate onto the cracker with the marshmallows. Put the remaining crackers on top to create 4 sandwiches. Wrap each one in the baking paper so it resembles a parcel. Cook in the fryer for 5 minutes at 340 F.

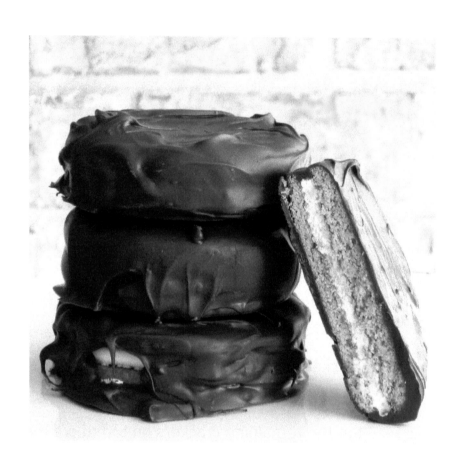

Apple Caramel Relish

Preparation Time: 40 min

Servings: 4

Nutrition Values: Calories: 382; Carbs: 56g; Fat: 18g; Protein: 3.4g

Ingredients

- 1 vanilla box cake
- 2 apples, peeled, sliced
- 3 oz butter, melted
- ½ cup brown sugar
- 1 tsp cinnamon
- ½ cup flour
- 1 cup caramel sauce

Directions

1. Line a cake tin with baking paper. In a bowl, mix butter, sugar, cinnamon and flour until you obtain a crumbly texture. Prepare the cake mix according to the instructions -no baking. Pour the batter into the tin and

arrange the apple slices on top. Spoon the caramel over the apples and add the crumble over the sauce. Cook in the Air fryer for 35 minutes at 360 F; make sure to check it halfway through, so it's not overcooked.

Chocolate and Peanut Butter Fondants

Preparation Time: 25 minutes

Servings: 4

Nutrition Values: Calories: 157; Carbs: 4g; Fat: 4g; Protein: 0.9g

Ingredients

- ¾ cup dark chocolate
- ½ cup peanut butter, crunchy
- 2 tbsp butter, diced
- ¼ cup + ¼ cup sugar
- 4 eggs, room temperature
- ⅛ cup flour, sieved
- 1 tsp salt
- ¼ cup water
- Cooking spray

Directions

1. Make a salted praline to top the chocolate fondant. Add ¼ cup of sugar, 1 tsp of salt

and water into a saucepan. Stir and bring it to a boil over low heat on a stove top. Simmer until the desired color is achieved and reduced.

2. Pour it into a baking tray and leave to cool and harden. Preheat the Air Fryer to 300 F. Place a pot of water over medium heat and place a heatproof bowl over it. Add the chocolate, butter, and peanut butter to the bowl.

3. Stir continuously until fully melted, combined, and smooth. Remove the bowl from the heat and allow to cool slightly. Add the eggs to the chocolate and whisk. Add the flour and remaining sugar; mix well.

4. Grease 4 small loaf pans with cooking spray and divide the chocolate mixture between them. Place 2 pans at a time in the basket and cook for 7 minutes. Remove them and

serve the fondants with a piece of salted praline.

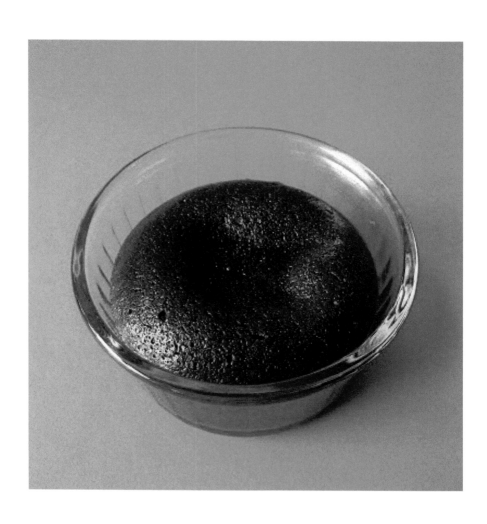

White Chocolate Pudding

Preparation Time: 40 min

Servings: 2

Nutrition Values: Calories : 320; Carbs: 3.06g;

Fat: 25g; Protein: 11g

Ingredients

- 3 oz white chocolate

- 4 large egg whites

- 2 large egg yolks, at room temperature

- ¼ cup sugar + more for garnishing

- 1 tbsp melted butter

- 1 tbsp unmelted butter

- ¼ tsp vanilla extract

- 1 ½ tbsp flour

Directions

1. Coat two 6-oz ramekins with melted butter. Add the sugar and swirl it in the ramekins to coat the butter. Pour out the remaining sugar and keep it. Melt the unmelted butter

with the chocolate in a microwave; set aside.

2. In another bowl, beat the egg yolks vigorously. Add the vanilla and kept sugar; beat to incorporate fully. Add the chocolate mixture and mix well. Add the flour and mix it with no lumps.

3. Preheat the Air Fryer to 330 F, and whisk the egg whites in another bowl till it holds stiff peaks. Add ⅓ of the egg whites into the chocolate mixture; fold in gently and evenly. Share the mixture into the ramekins with ½ inch space left at the top. Place the ramekins in the fryer basket, close the Air Fryer and cook for 14 minutes.

4. Dust with the remaining sugar and serve.

Lemon Curd

Preparation Time: 30 min

Servings: 2

Nutrition Values: Calories : 60; Carbs: 0g; Fat: 6g; Protein: 2g

Ingredients

- 3 tbsp butter
- 3 tbsp sugar
- 1 egg
- 1 egg yolk
- ¾ lemon, juiced

Directions

1. Add sugar and butter in a medium ramekin and beat evenly. Add egg and yolk slowly while still whisking. the fresh yellow color will be attained. Add the lemon juice and mix. Place the bowl in the fryer basket and cook at 250 F for 6 minutes. Increase the temperature again to 320 F and cook for 15 minutes.

2. Remove the bowl onto a flat surface; use a spoon to check for any lumps and remove. Cover the ramekin with a plastic wrap and refrigerate overnight or serve immediately.

Almond Meringue Cookies

Preparation Time: 145 min

Servings: 4

Nutrition Values: Calories : 215; Carbs: 35g; Fat: 1.6g; Protein: 7.6g

Ingredients

- 8 egg whites
- ½ tsp almond extract
- 1 ⅓ cups sugar
- ¼ tsp salt
- 2 tsp lemon juice
- 1 ½ tsp vanilla extract
- Melted dark chocolate to drizzle

Directions

1. In a mixing bowl, add egg whites, salt, and lemon juice. Beat using an electric mixer until foamy. Slowly add the sugar and continue beating until completely combined; add the almond and vanilla

extracts. Beat until stiff peaks form and glossy.

2. Line a round baking sheet with parchment paper. Fill a piping bag with the meringue mixture and pipe as many mounds on the baking sheet as you can leaving 2-inch spaces between each mound.

3. Place the baking sheet in the fryer basket and bake at 250 F for 5 minutes. Reduce the temperature to 220 F and bake for 15 more minutes. Then, reduce the temperature once more to 190 F and cook for 15 minutes. Remove the baking sheet and let the meringues cool for 2 hours. Drizzle with the dark chocolate before serving.

Chocolate Banana Sandwiches

Preparation Time: 30 min

Servings: 2

Nutrition Values: Calories: 240; Carbs: 26g; Fat: 9.1g; Protein: 12.3g

Ingredients

- 4 slices of brioche

- 1 tbsp butter, melted

- 6 oz milk chocolate, broken into chunks

- 1 banana, sliced

Directions

1. Brush the brioche slices with butter. Spread chocolate and banana on 2 brioche slices. Top with the remaining 2 slices to create 2 sandwiches. Arrange the sandwiches into your air fryer and cook for 14 minutes at 400 F, turning once halfway through. Slice in half and serve with vanilla ice cream.

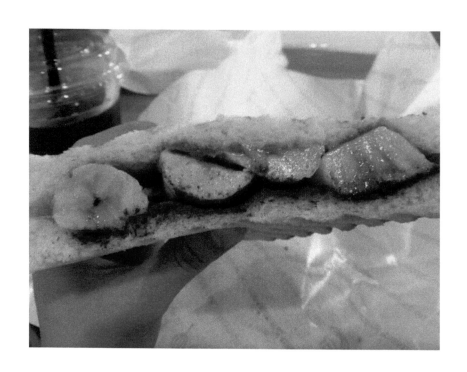

Crème Brulee

Preparation Time: 60 min

Servings: 3

Nutrition Values: Calories : 402; Carbs: 9.5g;
Fat: 32.5g; Protein: 13.6g

Ingredients

- 1 cup whipped cream
- 1 cup milk
- 2 vanilla pods
- 10 egg yolks
- 4 tbsp sugar + extra for topping

Directions

1. In a pan, add the milk and cream. Cut the vanilla pods open and scrape the seeds into the pan with the vanilla pods also. Place the pan over medium heat on a stove top until almost boiled while stirring regularly. Turn off the heat. Add the egg yolks to a bowl and beat it. Add the sugar and mix well but not too frothy.

2. Remove the vanilla pods from the milk mixture; pour the mixture onto the eggs mixture while stirring constantly. Let it sit for 25 minutes. Fill 2 to 3 ramekins with the mixture. Place the ramekins in the fryer basket and cook them at 190 F for 50 minutes. Once ready, remove the ramekins and let sit to cool. Sprinkle the remaining sugar over and use a torch to melt the sugar, so it browns at the top.

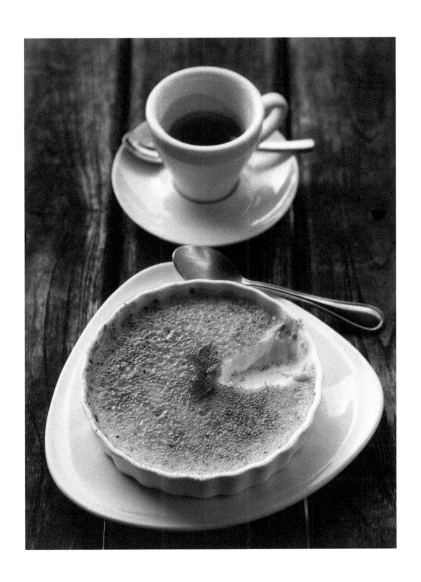

The Most Chocolaty Fudge

Preparation Time: 55 min

Servings: 8

Nutrition Values: Calories: 494; Carbs: 65.7g;

Fat: 25.1g; Protein: 5.6g

Ingredients

- 1 cup sugar

- 7 oz flour

- 1 tbsp honey

- ¼ cup milk

- 1 tsp vanilla extract

- 1 oz cocoa powder

- 2 eggs

- 4 oz butter

- 1 orange, juice and zest

- Icing:

- 1 oz butter, melted

- 4 oz powdered sugar

- 1 tbsp brown sugar

- 1 tbsp milk

- 2 tsp honey

Directions

1. Preheat the Air fryer to 350 F, and in a bowl, mix the dry ingredients for the fudge. Mix the wet ingredients separately; combine the two mixtures gently. Transfer the batter to a prepared cake pan. Cook for 35 minutes. Meanwhile whisk together all icing ingredients. When the cake cools, coat with the icing. Let set before slicing.